The Acupuncture Book

An Overview of the Benefits of Acupuncture

Acupuncture is an ancient healing method that can be used to compliment medicine as we know it in the western world today. Using the body's meridians, or energy lines, acupuncture stimulates the body to heal itself. It's not painful, there are no side effects, there is only balance and relaxation.

In this Itty Bitty® book you will learn about the major meridians of:

- Lung
- Heart or Pericardium – Circulatory System
- Kidneys
- Liver and Gall Bladder
- Gastro Intestinal System
- Digestive System

If you are interested in learning how acupuncture might benefit you and your health pick up a copy of this little book today.

Your Amazing Itty Bitty® Acupuncture Book

15 Steps that Answer Your Questions About the Art of Acupuncture

Yinjia "Rose" Gong, MD

Printed in the United States of America

Itty Bitty Publishing
311 Main Street, Suite D
El Segundo, CA 90245
(310) 640-8885

ISBN: 978-1-950326-23-5

This book has been written for people who
are interested in visiting an acupuncturist for
treatment and want to know more about
acupuncture. It is not a guide for using
acupuncture on yourself. Acupuncture should
only be practiced by trained acupuncturists.

This Book is dedicated to my dearest daughter Jenny who is always my biggest fan.

Stop by our Itty Bitty® website Directory to find to interesting information about acupuncture.

www.IttyBittyPublishing.com

Or visit my website at:

www.doc4pain.com

Table of Contents

Step 1.   Acupuncture Meridian Theory
Step 2.   Lung Meridian
Step 3.   Large Intestine Meridian
Step 4.   Stomach Meridian
Step 5.   Spleen Meridian
Step 6.   Heart Meridian
Step 7.   Small Intestine Meridian
Step 8.   Bladder Meridian
Step 9.   Kidney Meridian
Step 10.   Pericardium Meridian
Step 11.   San Jiao Meridian
Step 12.   Gall Bladder Meridian
Step 13.   Liver Meridian
Step 14.   Tips and Technics
Step 15.   Art, Philosophy and Circle of Life

Introduction

Many people have come to me over the years asking for details about acupuncture. Common questions are: Does it work? If so, how does it work? Can it be used to treat my condition?

My first impulse is to begin bringing up everything from the five years of traditional Chinese medicine theory I learned in medical school and from my long experience as a practitioner. Chinese medicine is quite involved, and very boring to learn, and when I try to explain it to people in great detail, I can see their eyes glaze over.

This is why I decided to write this book for people who want to lean how to take good care of their general health and have become curious about acupuncture.

If you are considering acupuncture you first want to be assured that acupuncture works. You want to know how it works and what it treats, and why you might want to consider it.

For prospective patients, I have created this as a guide to answering those questions. This as not a guide for performing acupuncture on yourself, but rather an overview of how acupuncture can benefit you or people you know and love.

Step 1.
Meridian Theory of Acupuncture

In this Itty Bitty Book, you will learn about the
12 acupuncture meridians. Most acupuncture
points are located on these meridians. You can't
see them or feel them. Doctors have tried to
prove their existence but have failed, and many
people doubt their existence. Can you say it exists
if you can't see it or feel it? What about Wi-Fi?
Can you see it? Can you touch it?

1. These meridians regulate energy flow
   and blood flow. The "traffic" along these
   pathways through the body is caused by
   blockages.
2. Acupuncture is like a traffic controller
   that allows the roads to clear. When it's
   done right, relief is the outcome.
3. From head to toe, acupuncture can
   alleviate most symptoms, whether you
   have a headache or neuropathic pain on
   your feet as long as you are on the right
   meridian you can fix the problem.
4. Good acupuncture should be able to
   relieve most symptoms within the first 5-
   minutes.

Meridian, Meridian, Meridian!

- It is not necessary to memorize the names of each acupuncture point. Instead, you simply master the meridians on which the points lie.
- Stimulating points along the meridian can remove blockages and help with conditions in the parts of body through which the meridian passes.
- If you have difficulty memorizing the meridian diagram, I have provided a website link to the meridian diagrams. Just go to:
  www.doc4pain.com/acupuncture, scroll down to the end, you will find the 12 meridian diagrams.
- Stay on the meridian, you wont get lost!
- Remember cross-treatment is more effective than same-side-treatment. For example, right side toothache can be treated from a left side hand point (Large Intestine Meridian).
- Look for points far from the affected area. Right side neck pain can be treated from left side arm points (San Jiao Meridian).
- Bloodletting is fast and effective in treating difficult cases. Again, stay on the meridian to blood let.
- Remember same side bloodletting works better than crossing.

Step 2.
Lung Meridian

In this chapter you will learn the pathway and functions of the lung meridian, and how you can apply this to treat illness. First of all, please have the lung meridian diagram in front of you. If you don't have it, then go to:

www.doc4pain.com/acupuncture.

Scroll down to the end, you will find 12 meridian diagrams. In this chapter I only explain the surface pathway, into which the needles will be put.

1. It starts at the front of the shoulder.
2. Down to anterior aspect of the arm.
3. Reach outside of the biceps.
4. Down to the base of the thumb.
5. Finish at the corner of the thumbnail.
6. Basically, by putting needles along this meridian, you can treat airway-associated diseases, such as sore throat and asthma.

Airway, Airway, Airway!

Understanding the Lung Meridian can be life saving, when someone is suffering from acute asthma who is far from a medical facility. It opens the airway instantly. Can't swallow because of sore throat? Blood let a couple of drops at the corner of your thumbnail. You will see an immediate effect. The following are key points on the lung meridian used to treat airway illnesses.

- Sore throat – LU1
- Asthma – LU2
- Pneumonia – LU5
- Cough – LU6
- Coughing up blood – LU6

Step 3
Large Intestine Meridian

Again, you don't have to memorize the Large Intestine Meridian diagram. Instead, go to: www.doc4pain.com/acupuncture, scroll down to find the Large Intestine Meridian. The surface pathway of the Large Intestine Meridian is as follows.

1. It begins at the outside corner of the index fingernail
2. Edge of the finger
3. Between the two tendons of the thumb at the wrist joint
4. Along the outer edge of the arm to the elbow
5. Outside of the elbow crease
6. Up the side of the neck
7. To the cheek
8. The lower gums
9. Top lip
10. Ending at the opposite nostril

Do You Suffer from Head and Facial Pain? Look for:

LI-4 (He Gu). Other points have similar effects, yet this point is used most frequently. The meridian goes to all the way to the head. So it treats many problems all over the head. It is a large intestine meridian so it alleviates some GI symptoms

- Headache
- Toothache
- Facial nerve paralysis
- Nose bleed
- Eye strain
- Sore throat
- Constipation
- Abdominal pain
- DO NOT use it in pregnant woman, it contracts the uterus.

Step 4
Stomach Meridian

Pathway of Stomach Meridian: For diagram, please go to: www.doc4pain.com/acupuncture, scroll down to find the stomach meridian.

1. Starts just below the eye.
2. Upper gum around the mouth.
3. Lower gum – in front of the ear – forehead.
4. Jaw – throat – collarbone.
5. Down to the lower abdomen – pubic area.
6. Anterior thigh – outside of kneecap.
7. Leg beside the shinbone,
8. Ending on the outside of the second toe.

Longevity, Weight Loss, and Rejuvenation Point

Is Zusanli (ST 36)

- This is a point that boosts your immune system; it is also called the longevity point.
- It rejuvenates you. Frequently putting pressure on this point makes you look younger and stronger.
- It alleviates most digestive system symptoms and illness.
- It is widely used in weight control, hypertension and diabetes.
- Many stroke patients benefit from using this point.
- This is a point you must learn before you learn any other points.
- You can use it for preventive care of the illnesses mentioned above.
- It is probably better than taking many supplements.
- This is the most important point of all acupuncture points!

Step 5
Spleen Meridian

Find the spleen meridian at:

www.doc4pain.com/acupuncture,

Scroll down to the end, find the diagram. Here is the surface pathway.

1. Starts on the inside tip of the big toe.
2. Inner aspect of the foot to the arch.
3. In front of the inner ankle.
4. Up the leg, just behind the bone.
5. Cross the knee- inner border of the kneecap.
6. Anterior thigh – groin.
7. Lower abdomen – in front of the shoulder.
8. Down to the axillary.

Meridian of Reproductive System

This is the meridian mainly used to treat reproductive problems for men and women. It also addresses some digestive symptom problems. The main point of this meridian is Sanyinjiao (SP6). It treats the following medical problems.

- Irregular menstrual period.
- Infertility.
- Impotence.
- Spermatorrhea.
- Enuresis.
- Swelling.
- Insomnia.
- Stomach pain.

Step 6
Heart Meridian

Looking at the diagram, you can see that the heart meridian is short on the body surface. Go to www.doc4pain.com/acupuncture to locate the diagram. Once you master this short version, you are on the right track. The pathway is as follows.

1. It surfaces around the inner aspect of the arm.
2. The inner end of the elbow crease.
3. The tip of the little finger by the corner of the nail on the thumb side.

Heart, Mind and Body

"The heart is the sovereign of all the organs and represents the consciousness of one's being. It is responsible for intelligence, wisdom and spiritual transformation."

~Yellow Emperor's
Classic of Medicine

The famous point of this meridian is Shenmen (HT7). It treats the following conditions

- Anxiety.
- Insomnia.
- Panic attack.
- Chest pain.
- Seizure.

Step 7
Small Intestine Meridian

Again, locate the surface small intestine meridian from www.doc4pain.com/acupuncture. Look for the solid line only. The surface pathway of the small intestine meridian is as follows:

1. Starts at corner of the little fingernail.
2. Edge of the hand to the wrist,
3. Flows up the forearm,
4. Outer edge of the (ulna) bone,
5. Back of the arm,
6. Behind the shoulder joint,
7. To the hollow above the collarbone,
8. Behind the muscle on the side of the neck,
9. Over the cheek to the ear.

Small Intestine Meridian – From Pinky to the Ear

The rule of thumb is that you can treat parts of body through which each specific meridian passes. The specific point in this meridian is Houxi (SI 3). Along the small intestine pathway, it treats the following illnesses.

- Ear problems
- Sore throat
- Eye strain
- Neck pain/stiffness
- Finger and arm pain

As you can see, you don't need to memorize the acupuncture points. All you need to do is to refer to the right meridian. Stay on the right meridian, you won't get lost.

Step 8
Bladder Meridian

This is the longest meridian in the body. Locate the meridian via:

www.doc4pain.com/acupuncture.

1. Begins at the inner corner of the eye.
2. Eyebrow over the forehead and skull.
3. Nape of the neck.
4. Base of the skull (occiput).
5. Divides into two branches that descend parallel with the spine.
6. Down the back of the thigh to the center of the knee-fold (Weizhong BL- 40).
7. To the center of the calf muscle.
8. Behind the outer ankle.
9. To the outer tip of the little toe.

Meridian of Your Back

This meridian mainly occupies your entire back. Obviously, it treats back pain. The acupuncture point to remember is Weizhong (BL- 40). It is located in the center of your knee fold. It treats the following illnesses:

- Back pain
- Spine pain

This chapter will serve the most important purpose if you are able to alleviate back pain within few minutes via blood letting (BL 40). Make sure blood-let is on the same side as the back pain. For example, left side of back pain, blood let left Weizhong (BL-40).

- How do you blood let? (First, you locate the area that you want to blood let. Then, find superficial vein around this area, use 25 G syringe needle to pock quickly and just deep enough to let the blood out. You need to blood-let out 0.5 to 2 ml of blood. Sometimes, just a few drops of blood will make significant difference. **Do not do this at home. Let your acupuncturist or doctor do it for you.**

Step 9
Kidney Meridian

The kidney meridian runs from the heart of the
sole of your foot to the collarbone. For the
diagram of the kidney meridian and the famous
acupuncture point of this meridian Taixi (KI 3),
please refer to www.doc4pain.com/acupuncture.
Scroll down to the end. Find the kidney meridian
and KI 3.

1. It begins under the little toe
2. The heart of the sole
3. Inner edge of the foot
4. Loops behind the inside ankle bone to the
   heel
5. Inner aspect of the leg
6. Calf and the inner thigh
7. Pubic area
8. Lower abdomen
9. To the collarbone

Kidney Meridian – Root of Life

In traditional Chinese medicine, the kidney meridian is considered to be the reservoir of energy. Taixi (KI3) is located at the indentation between medial malleolus and heel cord. It has many functions. The following is a summary of a few of them;

- Irregular menstrual period
- Impotence
- Frequent urination
- Insomnia
- Forgetfulness
- Hearing loss
- Tinnitus

Step 10
Pericardium Meridian

By now you are an expert in finding the diagram of this meridian. Here is the surface pathway.

1. It begins in the middle of the chest at the pericardium
2. Outside of nipple
3. Front of armpit
4. Down the arm
5. Through the biceps muscle
6. At the elbow crease it passes just to the inside of the biceps tendon
7. To the front of the forearm
8. To the wrist.
9. Ending in the outer corner of the middle fingernail.

Pericardium – Sack to protect the heart

This meridian guards the heart. Disruption of this meridian causes heart injury. It plays important roles in emotional states. It creates feelings of pleasure. The most important acupuncture point is Neiguan (PC6). It treats the following illnesses;

- Angina
- Palpitations
- Nausea/Vomiting
- Insomnia

Step 11
San Jiao Meridian

The San Jiao meridian is the only meridian in Chinese medicine that isn't associated with a western body organ.

1. It starts on the lateral corner of the ring finger nail
2. Up the forearm/up the triceps
3. Across the trapezium muscles
4. Around the ear
5. Ends at the outside of the eye

For the diagram of the San Jiao meridian, go to my website at www.doc4pain.com/acupuncture.

From the Ring Finger to the Side of The Head

From the Sanjiao meridian diagram (www.doc4pain.com/acupuncture), you can see it runs from ring finger to the side of head. So for headache, ear/eye problems, neck pain, look for points far from the affected areas – the ring finger and arm. Remember cross-treatment is more effective than the same-side-treatment. For right side headache, go to the left hand/arm.

The most important point that you have to remember is Waiguan (SJ 5). As with many points on this meridian, it treats the following:

- Headache
- Eye problems
- Ear problems
- Neck pain

I often use Waiguan (SJ 5) to treat neck pain. Relief comes within minutes!

Step 12
Gall Bladder Meridian

This meridian mainly runs from head to toe, along the side of body. For a detailed pathway, go to www.doc4pain.com/acupuncture.com.

1. It starts just outside of the outer corner of eye
2. Forehead just within the hairline
3. Behind the ear
4. Corner of the skull
5. Returns to the forehead above the center of eye
6. Contours the head to the bottom of skull
7. Down the neck behind the shoulder
8. Side of body behind the rib margin
9. Waist and pelvic crest
10. Down the outside of the leg
11. In front of the ankle
12. Ending on the outside of the 4th toe.

From Head to Toe, This Point Treats them All!

Rule of thumb, stimulating points along the meridian can remove the blockages and help with conditions in parts of body through which the meridian passes. Therefore, stimulating points along the gall bladder meridian can help with the following conditions:

- Eye problems
- Ear problems
- Neck pain
- Side of body problems, such as rib pain
- Low extremity problems – Hip pain, knee pain, ankle pain, and paralysis.
- Many points on this meridian can treat the conditions listed above. The most important point is Qiuxu (GB 40). I use this point often to treat rib pain or costochondritis. It relieves rib pain within 5-minutes!

Step 13
Liver Meridian

From the big toe to the rib, the liver meridian serves the area through which it passes. Any blockage of this meridian causes rib pain, lumbar pain, hernia, abdominal pain, inner thigh and foot problems. To find liver meridian diagram, please go to www.doc4pain.com/acupuncture, scroll down to the end.

1. Starts by the inside of the big toe
2. Top of toe
3. In front of inside ankle
4. Inner aspect of the leg
5. Inner thigh
6. Groin and pubic region
7. Lower abdomen – rib

The Spirits of Points – Liver Meridian

Besides treating the areas through which it passes, the liver meridian is also connected with the entire head including the face and brain (mood disorder). Therefore, it treats headaches, red eye and dry eye and mouth. It also treats mood disorder such as anger, depression and anxiety. Tai Chong (LR3) treats the following:

- Headache
- Dizziness
- Red eye
- Rib pain
- Seizure disorder
- Lower extremity paralysis
- Foot pain

Step 14
Tips and Technics

Acupuncture is "operator dependent" – meaning that treatment results can be different from one acupuncturist to another one. Therefore, learn the tips and technics to understand what your acupuncturist is doing. Your acupuncturist should:

1. Cross-treat. Locating the points across the body. For example, right side headache can be treated with left side hand points.
2. Locate the points far away from the affected area. For headaches, the acupuncturist should look for points in the hands or feet.
3. Blood-let whenever it is possible. Blood-let the same side. Blood-let far away from the affected area. It works wonders for some difficult cases. Your acupuncturist should look for tiny superficial veins to blood-let.
4. Looking for fast relief for acute pain management? No pain medications takes effect as fast as acupuncture.

More Tips and Techniques

- For chronic illness, your acupuncturist should keep the needles in at least 45-minutes or longer.
- For difficult cases, try blood letting first.
- Moving and exercising the affected area during acupuncture. For right shoulder pain, locate points at the left lower leg, move or exercise the right shoulder at the same time. This method is also called "Moving Qi" method.
- Synergy effect - put another needle near (1-2 inch) the main point aligned with the meridian. This will give synergic effect.
- When your method is working, use the same points. If it does not work during the first 3-visits, and then change the points.

Step 15
Art, Philosophy and Circle of Life

Each of the 12 main meridians has its own time to come to the forefront during every 24-hour period. It flows continuously, and the vital energy follows a specific timeline as it circulates through the body. Learn how these meridians work during their most effective times. When you follow the rhythm you improve your immune systems and healthy lifestyles. When you work against the flow, diseases start. The Table bellow shows these periods and associated meridians.

1.	Gallbladder	11 pm – 1 am
2.	Liver	1 am to 3 am
3.	Lung	3 am to 5 am
4.	Large Intestine	5 am to 7 am
5.	Stomach	7 am to 9 am
6.	Sleep	9 am to 11 am
7.	Heart	11 am to 1 pm
8.	Small Intestine	1 pm to 3 pm
9.	Bladder	3 pm to 5 pm
10.	Kidney	5 pm to 7 pm
11.	Pericardium	7 pm to 9 pm
12.	3 Jiao	9 pm to 11

24-Hour Cycle

- 11 pm to 3 am (Gallbladder and liver) you must get yourself into deep sleep during this time.
- 3 am to 5 am (Lung) daily deep breathing and white color food will help to nourish this meridian. If not, morning cough starts at 3 am.
- 5 am -7 am (Large intestine) – Time for bowel movement.
- 7 am to 9 am (Stomach) – Don't miss your breakfast!
- 9 am to 11 am (Spleen) – Spleen transports nutrients absorbed by stomach. If not, fatigue sinks in.
- 11 am to 1 pm (Heart) – Lunch and best time for 15 min nap.
- 1 pm to 3 pm (Small intestine) Absorb all your lunch and distribute everywhere in your body. Therefore high quality lunch is essential.
- 3 pm to 5 pm (Bladder) – Best time to nourish your bladder meridian by massaging the meridian.
- 5 pm to 7 pm (Kidney) – the most important organ in the Chinese medicine. Nourished with black color food, such as black bean, rice, and black mushroom.
- 7 pm to 9 pm (Pericardium) – Time for entertainment
- 9 pm to 11 pm (3 Jiao) – Sex time

You've finished. Before you go...

Tweet/share that you finished this book.

Please star rate this book.

Reviews are solid gold to writers. Please take a few minutes to give us some itty bitty feedback.

ABOUT THE AUTHOR

I graduated from Shanghai JiaoTong Medical School, formally Shanghai Second Medical University in Shanghai China. All physicians trained in China have to go through hundreds hours of Traditional Chinese Medicine training. This is to prepare all medical doctors to be able to combine Western Medicine and Traditional Chinese Medicine in their future practice.

After I came to the US, I went through many years of preparing for USMLE, internship and residency, today, I have been practicing pain management in California for over 20 years. With the opioid epidemic in the US, acupuncture is my first line of choice to manage pain.

Comparing to most of pain medications, acupuncture works faster and lasts longer. More importantly, it has no side effects and it treats the roots of the problem. With backgrounds both in Western and Traditional Chinese Medicine I differentiate myself from other pain doctors. I feel I am the most fortunate doctor in the world because my patients get better. Remember that the true wealth in this world is health.

If you enjoyed this book you might also like "Art of Acupuncture"

Other Itty Bitty® Books you might enjoy are:

- **Your Amazing Itty Bitty® Meditation Book** – Rhona Jordan

- **Your Amazing Itty Bitty® Self Esteem Book** – Jade Elizabeth

- **Your Amazing Itty Bitty® Heal Your Body Book** – Patricia Garza Pinto